Healthy K[barcode] Diet Cookbook

A Complete Ketogenic Diet Cookbook for Your Rapid Weight Loss and Lifelong Transformation

Lily Price

Disclaimer Notice:

Please note the information contained within this document is for educational and entertainment purposes only. All effort has been executed to present accurate, up to date, and reliable, complete information. No warranties of any kind are declared or implied. Readers acknowledge that the author is not engaging in the rendering of legal, financial, medical or professional advice. The content within this book has been derived from various sources. Please consult a licensed professional before attempting any techniques outlined in this book.

By reading this document, the reader agrees that under no circumstances is the author responsible for any losses, direct or indirect, which are incurred as a result of the use of information contained within this document, including, but not limited to, errors, omissions, or inaccuracies.

Table of Content

Introduction

Thank you for purchasing **Healthy Ketogenic Diet Cookbook: A Complete Ketogenic Diet Cookbook for Your Rapid Weight Loss and Lifelong Transformation** The ketogenic diet is a nutritional strategy based on the reduction of dietary carbohydrates, which "forces" the body to produce autonomously the glucose necessary for survival and to increase the energy consumption of fats contained in adipose tissue.

Ketogenic diet means "diet that produces ketone bodies" (a metabolic residue of energy production).

Regularly produced in minimal amounts and easily disposed of by urine and pulmonary ventilation, in the ketogenic diet ketone bodies reach a level above the normal condition. The undesirable excess of ketone bodies, responsible for the tendency to lower blood pH, is called ketosis.

BREAKFAST

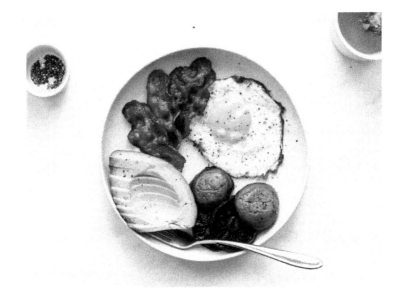

Fathead Bagels

Preparation Time: 20 minutes

Cooking Time: 15 minutes

Servings: 6

Ingredients:

- ¾ cup shredded mozzarella cheese

- 2 tablespoons cream cheese

- ¾ cup almond flour, plus additional as needed

- 1 large egg

- Salt

- Nonstick cooking spray

- 1 tablespoon Everything Bagel Seasoning

Directions:

1.	Preheat the oven to 400°F.

2.	In a microwave-safe bowl, add the mozzarella and cream cheese, and microwave on high for at least 1 minute. Stir the mixture then microwave again for 30 more seconds, until melted.

3.	Add the almond flour and egg, and season with salt. Mix everything together gently.

4.   When the dough is sticky, dust it with a little extra almond flour. Wrap the dough in plastic wrap and place it in the refrigerator for 10 minutes to firm up.

5.   Divide the dough into 6 balls and roll each out into a log.

6.   Spray a donut pan with cooking spray and wrap the dough around the tin's indentations. Top with the everything bagel seasoning.

7.   Bake the bagels for at least 15 minutes, until golden brown. Store leftovers in an airtight bag or container in the refrigerator for a week.

NUTRITION: Calories: 88 Total Fat: 7g Protein: 5g Total Carbs: 1g Fiber: 0g Net Carbs: 1g

Cheese Shell Breakfast Tacos

Preparation Time: 10 minutes

Cooking Time: 15 minutes

Servings: 2

Ingredients:

- 1⅓ cups shredded Mexican blend cheese

- 1 tablespoon butter or ghee

- 4 large eggs

- 2 tablespoons heavy whipping cream

- Salt

- Freshly ground black pepper

- Dash hot sauce

- 1 avocado, pitted, peeled, and sliced or cubed

- 1 tablespoon chopped cilantro

Directions:

1. Preheat the oven to 350°F. Line a baking sheet using a silicone baking mat or parchment paper.

2. Add ⅓-cup mounds of shredded cheese to the pan, leaving plenty of space between them. Bake until the each

sides are brown and the middle of each has fully melted, about 7 minutes.

3.   Set the pan on the cooking rack. You will need to move quickly to bend the shells while they are still pliable. You can get creative with what you want to bend them over. I like to create a "rack" over my sink with a wider cooling rack to drape them over or sometimes over the sides of a larger storage container. As they cool, they will harden.

4.   In a skillet, heat the butter at medium heat.

5.   Whisk in the eggs and heavy cream, and season with salt, pepper, and a dash of hot sauce.

6.   Scramble the eggs for 3 minutes, or to desired doneness.

7.   Fill the cheese shells with the scrambled eggs, and top with the avocado and cilantro.

Nutrition: Calories: 661 Total Fat: 57g Protein: 33g Total Carbs: 8g Fiber: 5g Net Carbs: 3g

Ham Spinach Ballet

Preparation Time: 10 minutes

Cooking time: 30 minutes

Servings: 2

Ingredients:

- 4 teaspoons cream

- ¾ pound fresh baby spinach

- 7-ounce ham, sliced

- Salt and black pepper, to taste

- 1 tablespoon unsalted butter, melted

Directions:

1. Set the oven to 360°F and grease 2 ramekins with butter.

2. Put butter and spinach in a skillet and cook for about 3 minutes.

3. Add cooked spinach in the ramekins and top with ham slices, cream, salt and black pepper.

4. Bake for about 25 minutes and dish out to serve hot.

5. For meal prepping, you can refrigerate this ham spinach ballet for about 3 days wrapped in a foil.

Nutrition: Calories: 188 Fat: 12.5g Carbs: 4.9g Protein: 14.6g

Sugar: 0.3g

KETO BREAD

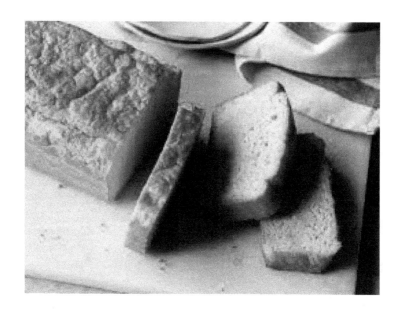

Keto Avocado Pancakes

Preparation Time: 5 minutes

Cooking Time: 10 minutes

Serves: 4

Ingredients:

- 1 Large Avocado

- 2 Eggs

- 1/2 cup Milk

- 1/4 cup Almond Flour

- 1/2 tsp. Baking Powder

- 1 tbsp. Erythritol

Directions:

1. Mix all ingredients in a blender.

2. Preheat a skillet and coat with non-stick spray.

3. Ladle in the batter and cook for 1-2 minutes per side.

Nutrition: Calories: 199 Fat: 16 g Protein: 7 g. Carbs: 4 g.

Keto Blueberry Bread

Preparation time: 10 minutes

Cooking time: 50 minutes

Servings: 8

Ingredients:

- 5 medium eggs
- 2 cups almond flour
- 2 tbsp. coconut flour
- 1/2 cup blueberries
- 1 1/2 tsp. baking powder
- 3 tbsp. heavy whipping cream
- 1/2 cup erythritol
- 3 tbsp. butter softened
- 1 tsp. vanilla extract

Directions:

1.   Whisk eggs with vanilla extract and sweetener in a large bowl using a hand mixer.

2.   Once it's frothy, add whipping cream and mix well.

3.   Separately, mix the dry and wet ingredients in two bowls then whisk them together.

4.   Add butter and beat well then fold in the berries.

5.   Slice and serve.

Nutrition: Calories 201 Fat 12.2 g Sodium 276 mg Carbs 4.3 g

Fiber 0.9 g Sugar 1.4 g

Keto Bread Twists

Preparation Time: 10 Minutes

Cooking Time: 20 Minutes

Servings: 10

Ingredients:

- 1/2 cup almond flour

- 4 tablespoons coconut flour

- 1/2 teaspoon salt

- 1 teaspoon baking powder

- 1 1/2 cups shredded cheese, preferably mozzarella

- 2/3 oz. butter

- 1 egg

- 2 oz. green pesto

- 1 egg, for brushing the top of the bread twists

Directions:

1.   Preheat the oven to 350°F.

2.   Mix all the dry ingredients in a bowl.

3.   Melt the butter and the cheese together on low heat. Stir with a wooden fork until the batter is smooth. Crack the egg and stir well.

4.   Add the dry ingredients and mix together into a firm dough.

5.   Place the dough between two sheets of parchment paper. Use a rolling pin and make a rectangle, about 1/5 inch thick.

6.   Remove the upper piece of parchment paper. Spread pesto on top and cut into 1-inch strips. Twist them and place on a baking sheet lined with parchment paper. Brush twists with the whisked egg.

7.   Bake in the oven for 15–20 minutes until they're golden brown.

Nutrition: Calories 204 Fat: 18g Protein: 7g Carbohydrates 3g Dietary Fiber 2g

Sesame Almond Crackers

Preparation Time: 10 minutes

Cooking Time: 24 minutes

Servings: 8

Ingredients:

- 8 Tbsp. unsalted butter, softened slightly

- 2 egg whites

- 1/2 tsp. salt

- 1/4 tsp. black pepper

- 2 1/4 cups almond flour

- 2 Tbsp. sesame seeds

Directions:

1. Preheat the oven to 350F.

2. Using a bowl, beat the egg whites, butter, salt, and black pepper.

3. Stir in the almond flour and sesame seeds.

4. Move the dough out between two pieces of parchment paper to a rectangle.

5. Peel off the top parchment paper and place the dough on a sheet pan.

6.   Cut the dough into crackers with a pizza cutter.

7.   Bake for 18 to 24 minutes, or until golden, rotating the

tray halfway through.

8.   Serve.

Nutrition: Calories: 299 Fat: 28g Carb: 4g Protein: 8g

Keto Fluffy Cloud Bread

Preparation Time: 25 minutes

Cooking time: 25 minutes

Servings: 3

Ingredients:

- pinch salt

- 1/2 Tbsp. ground psyllium husk powder

- 1/2 Tbsp. baking powder

- 1/4 tsp. cream of tarter

- eggs, separated

- 1/2 cup, cream cheese

Directions:

1. Preheat the oven at 300F and line a baking tray with parchment paper.

2. Whisk egg whites using a bowl.

3. Mix egg yolks with cream cheese, salt, cream of tartar, psyllium husk powder, and baking powder in a bowl.

4. Fold in the egg whites carefully and transfer to the baking tray.

5. Place in the oven and bake for 25 minutes.

6.   Remove from the oven and serve.

Nutrition: Calories: 185 Fat: 16.4g Carb: 3.9g Protein: 6.6

Keto Baguette Recipe

Preparation Time: 10 Minutes

Cooking Time: 45 Minutes

Servings: 3

Ingredients:

- 1/3 cup almond flour

- 1/4 cup psyllium husk powder

- 1/3 cup coconut flour

- 1/2 teaspoon baking soda

- 1 teaspoon salt

- 1 teaspoon xanthan gum

- Dry ingredients:

- 3 egg whites

- 1 whole egg

- 1/4 cup low-fat butter-milk

- 2 tablespoons Apple Cider Vinegar

- 1/3 cup lukewarm water

Directions::

1. Preheat the oven to 360°F. Mix all of the dry ingredients together into a bowl.

2.   In a different bowl, mix the buttermilk, egg whites and eggs together with an electric beater.

3.   Add the egg mixture to the dry ingredients and mix well using the same mixer until the dough is relatively thick. Add vinegar and lukewarm water and process until well combined.

4.   Using a spoon, scoop out sections and make a long baguette looking roll. You should be able to join together the different sections with your fingers.

5.   Place in the oven and cook for 10 minutes, then reduce the heat to 320°F and cook for another 30-40 mins. Cut and serve with olive oil and balsamic!

Nutrition: Calories 197 Total Fat 10g Protein 14g Fiber 3g Carbohydrates 5g

Sandwich Bread

Preparation Time: 30 minutes

Cooking time: 45 minutes

Servings: 20

Ingredients

- Avocado oil spray

- 2 cups almond flour

- 3/4 cup coconut flour

- 2 tablespoons psyllium husk powder

- 1 teaspoon salt

- 2 teaspoons baking powder

- 2 teaspoons instant yeast

- 2 tablespoons warm water

- 2 teaspoons coconut sugar

- 1 tablespoon beef gelatin

- 3 tablespoons plus 3/4 cup boiling water, divided

- 1 cup egg whites

- 2 tablespoons organic apple cider vinegar

- 5 drops liquid stevia

- 6 tablespoons ghee, melted and cooled slightly

- 1 teaspoon sesame seeds

Directions:

1.	Preheat the oven to 350F. Line the inside of a 9" × 5" loaf pan with parchment paper and lightly spray the inside with avocado oil.

2.	Merge together the almond flour, coconut flour, psyllium husk powder, salt, and baking powder.

3.	Merge together the yeast, warm water, and coconut sugar and let it sit 10 minutes until foamy.

4.	Whisk together the beef gelatin and 3 tablespoons boiling water until fully dissolved.

5.	In a medium bowl, stir together the dissolved yeast, dissolved gelatin, egg whites, vinegar, liquid stevia, and melted ghee.

6.	Whisk the dough into the prepared loaf pan and smooth out the top

7.	Bake about 75–90 minutes, covering the top with foil to prevent overbrowning if necessary.

8.	Let it cool before slicing.

Nutrition: Calories 197 Total Fat 10g Protein 14g Fiber 3g

Carbohydrates 5g

"Wheat" Bread

Preparation Time: 30 minutes

Cooking time: 45 minutes

Servings: 20

Ingredients

- 1/2 teaspoon instant yeast

- 1 tablespoon warm water

- 13/4 cups almond flour

- 4 tablespoons phylum husk powder

- 2 teaspoons baking powder

- 2 tablespoons raw sunflower seeds, coarsely chopped

- 4 teaspoons sesame seeds

- 2 teaspoons chia seeds

- 1 teaspoon salt

- 2 large eggs

- 4 large egg whites

- 2 tablespoons apple cider vinegar

- 10 drops liquid stevia

- 6 tablespoons butter

- 1/2 cup boiling water

Directions:

1.   Preheat the oven to 350F. Line the inside of a 9" × 5" loaf pan with parchment paper.

2.   Attach the yeast and warm water and stir to combine. Let it sit until foamy, about 5–10 minutes.

3.   Pour together the almond flour, psyllium husk powder, baking powder, sunflower seeds, sesame seeds, chia seeds, and salt.

4.   Pour together the eggs, egg whites, vinegar, liquid stevia, butter, and foamy yeast mixture.

5.   Bake until the loaf is golden brown

Nutrition: Calories 213 Total Fat 11 g Protein 14 g Fiber 2 g Carbohydrates 3 g

"White" Bread

Preparation Time: 13 minutes

Cooking time: 50 minutes

Servings: 10

Ingredients

- Avocado oil spray

- 1/2 teaspoon instant yeast

- 1 tablespoon warm water

- 6 large eggs

- 1/2 teaspoon cream of tartar

- 6 ounces cream cheese, softened slightly

- 2 tablespoons heavy whipping cream

- 1 teaspoon apple cider vinegar

- 5 drops liquid stevia

- 1/2 cup unflavored whey protein powder

- 1/2 tablespoon psyllium husk powder

- 1/4 teaspoon salt

- 1/4 teaspoon baking soda

Directions:

1.   Preheat the oven.

2.   Attach the yeast and warm water and stir to combine. Set aside until it's foamy, about 5–10 minutes.

3.   Attach the cream of tartar to the bowl with the egg whites.

4.   Attach the cream cheese, cream, vinegar, liquid stevia, and foamy yeast mixture to the bowl with the egg yolks.

5.   Pour the egg whites into the egg yolk mixture a little at a time, being careful not to deflate the whites

6.   Cool completely before slicing.

Nutrition: Calories 321 Total Fat 10 g Protein 12 g Fiber 2 g Carbohydrates 3 g

English Muffins

Preparation Time: 12 minutes

Cooking time: 50 minutes

Servings: 5

Ingredients

- 1 tablespoon unsaltcd butter, at room temperature

- 2 large eggs

- 4 tablespoons half-and-half

- 3 drops liquid stevia

- 6 tablespoons almond flour

- 4 tablespoons milled golden flaxseed

- 1 teaspoon baking powder

- 1/8 teaspoon salt

Directions:

1.	Preheat the oven to 350F. Spread the butter on the inside of four (1-cup) oven-safe ramekins. Cut four pieces of parchment paper to fit inside the bottom of each ramekin, and place each parchment paper circle inside.

2.	In a medium bowl, beat together the eggs, half-and-half, and liquid stevia.

3.   In a small bowl, whisk together the almond flour, flaxseed, baking powder, and salt.

4.   Stir the dry ingredients into the wet.

5.   Bake about 20–22 minutes.

6.   To remove the muffins, run a paring knife along the outside of each.

7.   To serve, slice each English Muffin in half across, and toast if desired.

Nutrition: Calories 143 Total Fat 9 g Protein 10 g Fiber 1 g Carbohydrates 3 g

Basic Biscuits

Preparation Time: 5 minutes

Cooking time: 1 hour

Servings: 8

Ingredients

- 1 cup almond flour

- 1 teaspoon baking powder

- 1/4 teaspoon salt

- 1/8 teaspoon black pepper

- 2 tablespoons chilled unsalted butter, diced

- 2 tablespoons heavy whipping cream

- 1 large egg

- 1/2 cup Cheddar cheese

Directions:

1.   Preheat the oven to 350F.

2.   Merge together the almond flour, baking powder, salt, and black pepper.

3.   Pour together the cream and egg, and gradually incorporate that into the almond flour mixture. Stir in the Cheddar until it's incorporated into the dough.

4.   Bake until golden on the bottom, about 20 minutes.

5.   Serve warm.

Nutrition: Calories 298 Total Fat 12 g Protein 11 g Fiber 3 g

Carbohydrates 3.3 g

Bagels

Preparation Time: 5 minutes

Cooking time: 1 hour

Servings: 8

Ingredients

- 1 teaspoon instant yeast

- 1 teaspoon coconut sugar

- 2 tablespoons warm water

- 1/2 teaspoon beef gelatin

- 2 tablespoons boiling water

- 1 cup almond flour

- 11/2 teaspoons psyllium husk powder

- 2 teaspoons baking powder

- 11/2 cups shredded low-moisture part-skim mozzarella

cheese

- 1 ounce cheese

- 1 large egg

- Avocado oil

- 1 large egg, lightly beaten with 1 tablespoon water, for egg wash
- 1 tablespoon everything bagel seasoning

Directions:

1. Preheat the oven to 400F.

2. In a small bowl, add the yeast, coconut sugar, and warm water and stir. Set aside until foamy, about 5–10 minutes.

3. Merge together the beef gelatin and boiling water.

4. Pour together the almond flour, psyllium husk powder, and baking powder and set aside.

5. Attach the mozzarella and cream cheese

6. Stir the yeast mixture and dissolved gelatin into the melted cheese until combined, then stir in the beaten egg.

7. Bake until golden on the bottom, about 12–14 minutes.

Nutrition: Calories 123 Total Fat 12 g Protein 9 g Fiber 4 g Carbohydrates 2.3 g

KETO PASTA

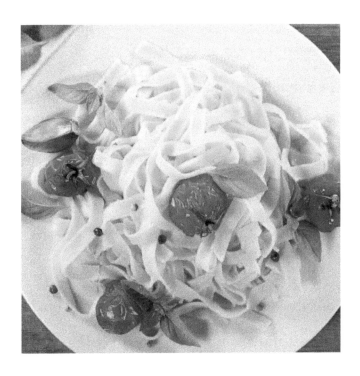

Tofu Avocado Keto Noodles

Preparation Time: 15 minutes

Cooking Time:30 minutes

Servings: 4

Ingredients:

• 2 tbsp. butter

• 1 lb. tofu

• Salt and black pepper to taste

• 8 large red and yellow bell peppers, Blade A, noodles trimmed

• 1 tsp. garlic powder

• 2 medium avocados, pitted, peeled and mashed

• 2 tbsp. chopped pecans for topping

Directions:

1. Melt the butter in a large skillet and cook the tofu until brown, 5 minutes. Season with salt and black pepper.

2. Merge in the bell peppers, garlic powder and cook until the peppers are slightly tender, 2 minutes.

3. Mix in the mashed avocados, adjust the taste with salt and black pepper and cook for 1 minute.

4.   Dish the food onto serving plates, garnish with the pecans and serve warm.

Nutrition: Calories: 209 Total Fat: 15.2g Saturated Fat: 7.3g Carbs: 5g Fiber: 1g, Sugar: 2g, Protein: 13g

Lemongrass Tempeh With Spaghetti Squash

Preparation Time:5 minutes

Cooking Time: 1 hour + 45 minutes marinating time

Servings: 4

Ingredients:

- For the lemongrass tempeh:

- 2 tbsp. minced lemongrass

- 2 tbsp. fresh ginger paste

- 2 tbsp. sugar-free maple syrup

- 2 tbsp. coconut aminos

- 1 tbsp. Himalayan salt

- 4 tempeh

- 2 tbsp. avocado oil

- For the squash noodles:

- 3 lb. spaghetti squashes, halved and deseeded

- 1 tbsp. olive oil

- Salt and black pepper to taste

- For the steamed spinach:

- 1 tbsp. avocado oil

- 1 tsp. fresh ginger paste

- 1 lb. baby spinach

- For the peanut-coconut sauce:

- 1/2 cup coconut milk

- 1/4 cup organic almond butter

Directions:

1. For the lemongrass tempeh:

2. In a medium bowl, mix the lemongrass, ginger paste, maple syrup, coconut aminos, and Himalayan salt. Place the tempeh in the liquid and coat well. Allow marinating for 45 minutes.

3. After, heat the avocado oil in a large skillet, remove the tempeh from the marinade and sear in the oil on both sides until golden brown and cooked through, 10 to 15 minutes

4. For the spaghetti squash:

5. Preheat the oven.

6. Place the spaghetti squashes on a baking sheet, brush with the olive oil and season with salt and black pepper. Bake in the oven for 20 to 25 minutes or until tender.

7. When ready, remove the squash and shred with two forks into spaghetti-like strands. Keep warm in the oven.

8. For the spinach:

9. In another skillet, heat the avocado oil and sauté the ginger until fragrant. Add the spinach and cook to wilt while stirring to be coated well in the ginger, 2 minutes. Turn the heat off.

10. For the almond-coconut sauce:

11. In a medium bowl, quickly whisk the coconut milk with the almond butter until well combined.

12. To serve:

13. Unwrap and divide the tempeh into four bowls, add the spaghetti squash to the side, then the spinach and drizzle the almond sauce on top.

14. Serve immediately.

Nutrition: Calories: 457, Total Fat: 37g Saturated Fat: 8.1g Total Carbs: 1.7g Fiber: 5g, Sugar: 4g, Protein: 22g

Chinese Seitan And Celeriac Noodles

Preparation Time: 10 minutes

Cooking Time: 1 hour 18 minutes

Servings: 4

Ingredients:

- 3 tbsp. sugar-free maple syrup

- 3 tbsp. coconut aminos

- 1 tbsp. fresh ginger paste

- 1/4 tsp. Chinese five spice powder

- Salt and black pepper to taste

- 1 lb. seitan, cut into 1-inch cubes

- 2 tbsp. butter

- 4 medium large celeriac, peeled and Blade B noodle
trimmed

- 1 tbsp. sesame oil

- 4 heads baby bok choy, leaves separated

- 2 green onions, chopped for garnishing

- 2 tbsp. sesame seeds for garnishing

Directions:

1.   Preheat the oven.

2.	In a large bowl, mix the maple syrup, coconut aminos, ginger paste, Chinese five-spice powder, salt, and black pepper. Spoon 3 tablespoons of the mixture into a small bowl and reserve for topping. Mix the seitan cubes into the remaining marinade and set aside to marinate for 25 minutes.

3.	Meanwhile, dissolve the butter in a medium skillet and sauté the celeriac until softened, 5 to 7 minutes or until tender. Turn the heat off and set aside.

4.	When the marinating is over, remove the seitan from the marinade onto the baking sheet and cook in the oven for 40 minutes or until cooked through.

5.	When the seitan is almost ready, heat the sesame oil in a large skillet and sauté the bok choy and zucchini pasta until slightly wilted and tender, 2 to 3 minutes.

6.	Drizzle the reserved marinade on top and serve warm.

Nutrition: Calories: 702, Total Fat: 54.9g, Total Carbs: 5g, Fiber: 1g, Sugar: 4g, Protein: 47g

Creamy Tuscan Tofu Linguine

Preparation Time: 12 minutes

Cooking Time: 35 minutes

Servings: 4

Ingredients:

- For the keto linguine:

- 1 cup shredded mozzarella cheese

- 1 egg yolk

- For the creamy Tuscan tofu:

- 2 tbsp. olive oil

- 4 tofu

- 1 medium white onion, chopped

- 1 cup tomatoes in oil,

- 1 red bell pepper, deseeded and chopped

- 5 garlic cloves, minced

- 1 tsp. dried oregano

- 3/4 cup vegetable broth

- 1 1/2 cup coconut cream

- 3/4 cup grated parmesan cheese

- 1 cup baby kale, chopped

- Salt and black pepper to taste

Directions:

1. For the keto linguine:

2. Pour the cheese into a medium safe-microwave bowl and melt in the microwave for 35 minutes or until melted.

3. Take out the bowl and allow cooling for 1 minute only to warm the cheese but not cool completely. Mix in the egg yolk until well-combined.

4. Lay a parchment paper on a flat surface, pour the cheese mixture on top and cover with another parchment paper.

1. When ready to cook, bring 2 cups of water to a boil in medium saucepan and add the keto linguine. Cook and then drain through a colander. Run cold water over the pasta and set aside to cool.

5. For the creamy Tuscan tofu:

6. Heat the olive oil in skillet, season the tofu with salt, black pepper, and cook in the oil until golden brown on the outside and cooked within, 7 to 8 minutes. Transfer the tofu to a plate and cut into 4 slices each. Set aside.

7. Add the onion, sundried tomatoes, bell pepper to the skillet and sauté until softened, 5 minutes. Mix in the garlic, oregano and cook until fragrant, 1 minute.

8. Deglaze the skillet with the vegetable broth and mix in the coconut cream. Simmer for 2 minutes and stir in the parmesan cheese until melted, 2 minutes.

9. Once the cheese melts, stir in the kale to wilt and adjust the taste with salt and black pepper.

10. Mix in the linguine and tofu until well coated in the sauce.

11. Dish the food and serve warm.

Nutrition: Calories: 127, Total Fat: 12.7g, Saturated Fat: 4.6g, Carbs: 1g, Fiber: 0g, Sugar: 0g, Protein: 3g,

One-Pot Spicy Cheddar Pasta

Preparation Time: 35 minutes

Cooking Time: 50 minutes

Servings: 4

Ingredients:

- For the shirataki fettuccine:

- 2 (8 oz.) packs shirataki fettuccine

- For the spicy cheddar pasta:

- 4 tempeh

- 1 medium yellow onion, minced

- 3 garlic cloves, minced

- 1 tsp. Italian seasoning

- 1/2 tsp. garlic powder

- 1/4 tsp. red chili flakes

- 1/4 tsp. cayenne pepper

- 1 cup sugar-free marinara sauce

- 1 cup grated mozzarella cheese

- 1/2 cup grated cheddar cheese

- Salt and black pepper to taste

- 2 tbsp. chopped parsley

Directions:

1.   For the shirataki fettuccine:

2.   Boil water .

3.   Strain the shirataki pasta through a colander and rinse very well under hot running water.

4.   Allow proper draining and pour the shirataki pasta into the boiling water. Cook for 3 minutes and strain again.

5.   Place a dry skillet over medium heat and stir-fry the shirataki pasta until visibly dry, and makes a squeaky sound when stirred, 1 to 2 minutes. Take off the heat and set aside.

6.   For the spicy cheddar pasta:

7.   Heat the olive, season the tempeh with salt, black pepper, and cook in the oil until golden brown on both sides and cooked within, 10 minutes. Transfer to a plate, cut into cubes and set aside.

8.   Attach the onion and garlic to the pan and cook, 3 minutes. Season with the Italian seasoning, garlic powder, red chili flakes, and cayenne pepper. Cook for 1 minute.

9.   Stir in the marinara sauce, cover the pot and simmer for 5 minutes. Open the lid and adjust the taste with salt and black pepper.

10.   Stir until the cheese melts.

11.   Dish the food onto serving plates and garnish with the parsley.

12.   Serve warm.

Nutrition: Calories: 208, Total Fat: 20g Carbs: 1g, Fiber: 0g, Sugar: 1g, Protein: 7g,

Mushroom Alfredo Zoodles

Preparation Time: 23 minutes

Cooking Time: 30 minutes

Servings: 4

Ingredients:

- 4 tbsp. butter

- 4 mushrooms, cut into 1-inch cubes

- Salt and black pepper to taste

- 4 large turnips, peeled and Blade C noodle trimmed

- 3 garlic cloves, minced

- 3/4 cup coconut cream

- 1 cup grated parmesan cheese

- 2 tbsp. chopped fresh parsley

Directions:

1. Dissolve the butter with salt, black pepper.

2. Dissolve the remaining butter and sauté the turnips until softened, 6 minutes.

3. Attach the garlic to the pan and cook until fragrant, 1 minute.

4. Reduce the heat to low and stir in the coconut cream and parmesan cheese until melted. Season with salt, black pepper.

5. Stir in the mushroom and dish the food onto serving plates.

6. Garnish with the parsley and serve warm.

Nutrition: Calories: 127, Total Fat: 12.7g, Carbs: 1g, Fiber: 0g, Sugar: 0g, Protein: 3g

Penne Alla Vodka

Preparation time: 5 minutes

Cooking Time: 35 minutes

Serving Size: 4

Ingredients:

• 1/2 cup heavy cream

• 1/2 cup (freshly grated) Parmesan

• 3 tablespoon butter

• Kosher salt

• 1 lb. tubed pasta

• 1 shallot (minced)

• 1/2 teaspoon (crushed) red pepper flakes

• 2 tablespoon vodka

• 2 cloves garlic (minced)

• 1/2 cup tomato paste

• Basil, for serving

Directions:

1. Melt the butter in a big saucepan over medium heat.

2. Include the shallot and garlic and simmer, constantly stirring, for four to five minutes, until tender.

3. Include the tomato sauce and red pepper and simmer for five minutes, frequently stirring, until the paste is filled with shallots and cloves and begins to darken.

4. Add vodka to the bowl and stir to mix it, removing from the bottom of the container some browned pieces. Turn the heat off.

5. Bring to a boil the big pot of salted water and prepare the pasta until it is al dente. Before draining, save two cups of pasta sauce.

6. Return the sauce to heat and add 1/4 cup of heavy cream and pasta liquid, stirring until mixed.

7. Insert half of the Parmesan cheese and mix until it has dissolved. Turn the heat off and add the cooked pasta.

8. If the sauce appears dry, add in the leftover Parmesan cheese and include more pasta water (about a tablespoons at the moment).

9. If required, sprinkle salt. With more Parmesan and shredded basil leaves, serve hot.

Nutrition: Calories 336 Fat 17g, Protein 38g, Sodium 692mg, Total Carbs 3g, Fiber 3g

Spinach Lamb Whole Wheat Pasta

Preparation Time: 5 minutes

Cooking time: 25–30 minutes

Servings: 5

Ingredients

- 6 cups chopped spinach

- 1/2 pound whole-wheat elbow noodles

- 1 pound ground lamb

- 1 (14-ounce) can unsalted diced tomatoes

- 1 medium onion, chopped

- 4 cloves garlic, thinly sliced

- 2 tablespoons tahini paste

- 1 teaspoon dried oregano

- 1 teaspoon ground cumin

- 3/4 teaspoon salt

- 1 quart water

- 2 tablespoons crumbled feta cheese

Directions

1. To a large cooking pot, add the lamb, pasta, tahini, spinach, onion, tomatoes, garlic, cumin, oregano and salt.

2.   Stir in the water and heat over medium-high heat.

3.   Allow the pasta mixture to boil gradually.

4.   Cook the mixture, stirring periodically, until the pasta is cooked to your satisfaction, about 10–12 minutes.

5.   Take the pasta mixture off the heat.

6.   Top with the feta cheese and serve warm.

Nutrition: Calories 400 Fat 16 g Carbs 4.2 g Protein 24 g Sodium 444 mg

Bacon Whole Wheat Pasta

Preparation Time: 5 minutes

Cooking time: 15 minutes

Servings: 4

Ingredients

- 3 strips bacon, preferably thick cut

- 1/2 pound whole wheat pasta

- 2 cups water or broth

- 2 cloves garlic, minced

- 1/3 cup crumbled blue cheese

- 1/4 cup chopped sun dried tomatoes

- 2 tablespoons milk

- Walnuts and parsley (optional, for garnishing)

Directions

1. To a large skillet or saucepan, add the bacon and cook over medium-high heat until crispy. Set aside half the cooked bacon, drain on paper towels and crumble.

2. Break the remaining bacon into chunks; stir in the pasta, water, garlic or broth, and tomatoes.

3. Cover and boil the mixture.

4.   Allow the mixture to simmer for 7–8 minutes, until the pasta is cooked to your satisfaction.

5.   Take the pasta mixture off the heat and mix in the milk and cheese. Combine until the cheese melts.

6.   Top with the reserved bacon, walnuts and parsley and serve warm.

Nutrition: Calories 504 Fat 9 g Carbs 4 g Protein 22 g Sodium 274 mg

Tomato Lamb Gemelli

Preparation Time: 5 minutes

Cooking time: 35–40 minutes

Servings: 6

Ingredients

- 1 tablespoon olive oil

- 1 medium onion, chopped

- 2 cloves garlic, minced

- 15 ounces ground lamb

- 3 tablespoons tomato paste

- 1 teaspoon salt

- 1/4 teaspoon red chili flakes

- 1 tablespoon fresh rosemary, chopped

- 3 cups tomatoes, diced

- 2 cups unsalted beef or chicken broth

- 31/2 cups gemelli or other small pasta

Directions

1. Add the oil to a large cooking pot and heat it over medium heat.

2.   Add the onions and garlic and sauté while stirring until softened, about 3–4 minutes.

3.   Increase the heat and mix in the lamb. Break it into small pieces. Stir-cook until lightly browned, about 5–7 minutes.

4.   Mix in the tomato paste, rosemary, salt and pepper flakes; stir-cook for 2 minutes. Stir in the broth and tomatoes; allow the mixture to boil gradually.

5.   Turn down heat to low. Allow the mixture to simmer for 14–15 minutes.

6.   Mix in the pasta and boil the mixture.

7.   Allow the mixture to simmer for 10 minutes, until the pasta is cooked to your satisfaction.

8.   Serve warm.

Nutrition: Calories 383 Fat 14 g Carbs 4.2 g Protein 21 g Sodium 486 mg

KETO CHAFFLE

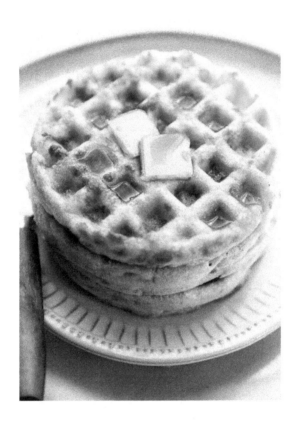

Basic Sweet Chaffle

Preparation time: 5 minutes

Cooking time: 15 minutes

Servings: 2

Ingredients

- Egg (1)

- Shredded mozzarella cheese (.5 cup)

- Swerve Brown Sweetener (2 tbsp.)

- Cinnamon (.5 tsp.)

Directions:

1. Preheat the mini waffle iron.

2. Whip the eggs using a fork and add in the cheese.

3. Pour half of the mixture into the waffle maker and cook it until it's golden brown (4 min.).

4. In another mixing bowl, whisk the cinnamon and Swerve Brown Sweetener.

5. Once the chaffle is done, cut it into slices while it's still hot and add it to the cinnamon mixture. It soaks up more of the mix when it's still hot!

6. Serve it piping hot.

Nutritiona: Carbohydrates: 2.9 Calories: 76 Protein: 5.5 grams

Fats: 4.3 grams

Carnivore Chaffle

Preparation time: 5 minutes

Cooking time: 15 minutes

Servings: 2

Ingredients

- Ground pork rinds (.5 cup)

- Shredded cheddar cheese (.33 cup)

- Egg (1 lightly whisked)

- Salt (1 pinch)

Directions:

1. Warm a mini-waffle iron and spritz it with a spritz of cooking oil.

2. Whisk the cheese, egg, salt, and rinds in a mixing container.

3. Dump the batter into the waffle maker in two batches to cook for five minutes. Serve and garnish as desired.

Nutrition: Carbohydrates: 0.8 grams Calories: 275 Protein: 23.6 grams Fats: 20.2 grams

Cauliflower Chaffles

Preparation time: 5 minutes

Cooking time: 15 minutes

Servings: 2

Ingredients

• Riced cauliflower (1 cup)

• Garlic powder (.25 tsp.)

• Ground black pepper (.25 tsp.)

• Italian seasoning (.5 tsp.)

• Salt (.25 tsp.)

• Shredded mozzarella/Mexican blend cheese (.5 cup)

• Egg (1)

• Shredded parmesan cheese (.5 cup)

Directions:

1. Toss each of the fixings into a blender. Sprinkle 1/8 cup of parmesan in the waffle iron, entirely covering the base.

2. Fill it with the cauliflower mix with a sprinkle of parmesan on top.

3. Cook until crispy or about four to five minutes.

4. Serve now or freeze them for later.

Nutrition: Carbohydrates: 5 grams Calories: 246 Protein: 20 grams Fats: 16 grams

Cream Cheese Mini Chaffles

Preparation time: 5 minutes

Cooking time: 15 minutes

Servings: 2

Ingredients

- Coconut flour (2 tsp.)

- Monk fruit/Swerve (4 tsp.)

- Baking powder (.25 tsp.)

- Unchilled whole egg (1)

- Unchilled cream cheese (1 oz.)

- Vanilla extract (.5 tsp.)

Directions:

1. Dump the cold eggs into warm water for three to five minutes to remove the chill. Place the cream cheese in a microwave-safe dish and cook it for 15 seconds or until it's softened in the microwave.

2. Warm the grill as you wait.

3. Whisk the swerve, baking powder, and flour. Mix in the cream cheese, egg, and vanilla extract.

4.   Pour the batter into the iron for three to four minutes.

Top it off as desired.

Nutrition: Carbohydrates: 2.4 grams Protein: 5 grams Fats:

8.3 grams

Jalapeno Bacon Chaffle

Preparation time: 5 minutes

Cooking time: 30 minutes

Servings: 2

Ingredients

- Eggs (4)

- Cheddar cheese - shredded (2 cups)

- Freshly chopped chives (1 tbsp. + more for garnish)

- Softened cream cheese (.5 cup)

- Garlic cloves (.5 tsp.)

- Scallion (1)

- Bacon - chopped and cooked (.5 cup)

- Fresh jalapeños - seeded (2)

- Scallion (half of 1 - for garnish)

Directions:

1.   Warm and lightly grease the waffle maker.

2.   Mince the garlic, scallion, chives, and jalapenos.

3.   Toss all of the fixings into a mixing bowl and beat to combine.

4.   Evenly spoon the mixture over the bottom plate, spreading it out slightly to get an even result.

5.   Close the waffle iron and cook for about six minutes, depending on your waffle maker.

6.   Mix the cream cheese, garlic, and spring onions into a bowl and beat well to combine. Add most of the bacon, retaining some for garnish, and stir thoroughly.

7.   Gently lift the lid when you think they're done.

8.   Top them off using a big spoonful of cream cheese, sliced jalapeño, the remaining chopped chives, and bacon.

Nutrition: Carbohydrates: 4 grams Calories: 399 Protein: 21 grams Fats: 33 grams

Keto Sandwich Chaffle

Preparation time: 5 minutes

Cooking time: 30 minutes

Servings: 2

Ingredients

- Eggs (2 large)

- Superfine blanched almond flour (.25 cup)

- Garlic powder (.5 tsp.)

- Baking powder (.75 tsp.)

- Shredded cheese (1 cup)

- Your favorite nitrate-free deli meat, turkey, ham, chicken (3 slices)

- Cooked bacon (2 slices)

- Tomatoes (2 slices)

- Cheddar cheese (1 slice)

- Keto-friendly chicken salad (.25 cup)

- Keto-friendly tuna salad (.25 cup)

- Also Needed: Dash Mini-Waffle Maker/Belgian Waffle Maker

Directions:

1.   Set the waffle iron on the high setting to heat and spritz with a cooking oil spray.

2.   Whisk the eggs, flour, garlic powder, and baking powder, mixing in the cheese last.

3.   Pour 1/4 cup of batter into the waffle maker and close the lid.

4.   Note: If you're using a Belgian waffle maker, pour half of the batter into the middle of the iron and close the lid. Cook until crispy, flip it over and continue cooking until it's browned.

5.   Finish the batter using the same process.

6.   Serve using your favorite sandwich fillings.

Nutrition: Carbohydrates: 3 grams Calories: 202 Protein: 14 grams Fats: 15 grams

MAIN, SIDE & VEGETABLE

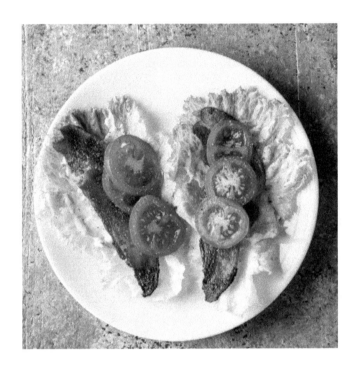

Blackened Chicken

Preparation time: 10 minutes

Cooking time: 10 minutes

Servings: 2

Ingredients:

- 1/4 teaspoon paprika

- 1/8 teaspoon salt

- ¼ teaspoon cayenne pepper

- ¼ teaspoon ground cumin

- ¼ teaspoon dried thyme

- 1/8 teaspoon ground white pepper

- 1/8 teaspoon onion powder

- chicken breast, boneless and skinless

Directions:

1.   Preheat your oven to 350 degrees Fahrenheit. Grease baking sheet. Take a cast-iron skillet and place it over high heat.

2.   Add oil and heat it for 5 minutes until smoking hot.

3.   Take a small bowl and mix salt, paprika, cumin, white pepper, cayenne, thyme, onion powder. Oil the chicken breast on both sides and coat the breast with the spice mix.

4.   Transfer to your hot pan and cook for 1 minute per side.

5.   Transfer to your prepared baking sheet and bake for 5 minutes.

6.   Serve and enjoy!

Nutrition: Calories: 136 Fat,: 3g Carbohydrates: 2g Protein: 24g Fiber: 1g Net Carbohydrates: 1g

Mediterranean Mushroom Olive Steak

Preparation time: 10 minutes

Cooking time: 14 minutes

Servings: 2

Ingredients:

• 1/2 pound boneless beef sirloin steak, ¾ inch thick, cut into 4 pieces

• 1/2 large red onion, chopped

• 1/2 cup mushrooms

• 2 garlic cloves, thinly sliced

• 2 tablespoons olive oil

• 1/4 cup green olives, coarsely chopped

• 1/2 cup parsley leaves, finely cut

Directions:

1. Take a large-sized skillet and place it over medium-high heat.

2.   Add oil and let it heat up. Add beef and cook until both sides are browned, remove beef and drain fat. Add the rest of the oil to the skillet and heat it.

3.   Add onions, garlic, and cook for 2-3 minutes. Stir well.

4.   Add mushrooms olives and cook until mushrooms are thoroughly done. Return beef to skillet and lower heat to medium.

5.   Cook for 3-4 minutes (covered). Stir in parsley.

6.   Serve and enjoy!

Nutrition: Calories: 386 Fat,: 30g Carbohydrates: 11g Protein: 21g Fiber: 5g Net Carbohydrates: 6g

Super Bowl with Eggplant and Chicken

Preparation Time: 3 minutes

Cooking Time: 8 minutes

Servings: 4

Ingredients:

- tablespoon olive oil

- leek, chopped

- chicken breasts, diced

- pound eggplant, peeled and sliced

- 1 teaspoon garlic paste

- 1/2 teaspoon turmeric powder

- 1 teaspoon red pepper flakes

- 1 cup broth, preferably homemade

- 1 cup tomatoes, puréed

- Kosher salt and ground black pepper, to taste

Directions:

1. Press the "Sauté" button to heat up your Instant Pot.
Then, heat the oil. Cook the leeks until softened.

2.   Now, add the chicken breasts; cook for 3 to 4 minute or until they are no longer pink. Then, add the remaining ingredients; stir to combine well.

3.   Secure the lid. Choose "Poultry" mode and High pressure; cook for 5 minutes. Once cooking is complete, use a natural pressure release; carefully remove the lid.

4.   Divide your dish among serving bowls and serve warm. Bon appétit!

Nutrition: 317 Calories; 20.9g Fat; 6.4g Total Carbs; 22.9g Protein; 3.8g Sugars

Warm Chinese-Style Salad

Preparation Time: 2 minutes

Cooking Time: 8 minutes

Servings: 4

Ingredients:

- 2 tablespoons sesame oil

- yellow onion, chopped

- teaspoon garlic, finely minced

- pound pe-tsai cabbage, shredded

- 1/4 cup rice wine vinegar

- 1/4 teaspoon Szechuan pepper

- 1/2 teaspoon salt

- 1 tablespoon soy sauce

Directions:

1. Press the "Sauté" button to heat up your Instant Pot. Then, heat the sesame oil. Cook the onion until softened.

2. Add the remaining ingredients.

3. Secure the lid. Choose "Manual" mode and High pressure; cook for 3 minutes. Once cooking is complete, use a quick pressure release; carefully remove the lid.

4.   Transfer the cabbage mixture to a nice salad bowl and serve immediately. Enjoy!

Nutrition: 116 Calories; 7.7g Fat; 6.2g Total Carbs; 2.1g Protein; 3.3g Sugars

Squash Wedges

Preparation Time: 10 minutes

Cooking Time: 10 minutes

Servings: 4

Ingredients:

- pound butternut squash, cut into medium wedges
- Olive oil for frying
- A pinch of salt and black pepper
- ¼ teaspoon baking soda

Directions:

1. Heat a pan with olive oil at medium-high heat, put squash wedges, season with salt, pepper and the baking soda, cook until they are gold on all sides, drain grease, divide between plates then serve.

Nutrition: Calories: 202 Fat: 5 Fiber: 5 Carbs: 7 Protein: 11

Jalapeno and Cheese Egg Muffins

Preparation time: 10 minutes

Cooking time: 15 minutes

Servings: 2

Ingredients:

- jalapeno pepper, diced

- tbsp sliced green onions

- tbsp grated parmesan cheese

- tsp all-purpose seasoning

- eggs

- Seasoning:

- 1/3 tsp salt

- ¼ tsp ground black pepper

Directions:

1. Turn on the oven, then set it to 375 degrees F, and let it preheat.

2. Meanwhile, take two silicone muffin cups, grease with oil, and evenly fill them with cheese, jalapeno pepper, and green onion.

3.   Crack eggs in a bowl, season with salt, black pepper, and all-purpose seasoning, whisk well, then evenly pour the mixture into muffin cups and bake for 15 to 20 minutes or until the top is slightly brown and muffins have puffed up.

4.   Serve.

Nutrition: 108 Calories; 7.1 g Fats; 8.9 g Protein; 1.8 g Net Carb; 0.4 g Fiber;

Cheesy Tomato and Olive Muffins

Preparation time: 10 minutes

Cooking time: 12 minutes

Servings: 2

Ingredients:

- 4 1/3 tbsp almond flour

- ½ tbsp coconut flour

- 1/3 tbsp chopped tomato

- 1/3 tbsp sliced green olives

- 2 tbsp sour cream

- Seasoning:

- 1/8 tsp baking powder

- 2/3 tbsp avocado oil

- 3 tbsp grated parmesan cheese

- ½ of egg

Directions:

1. Turn on the oven, then set it to 320 degrees F and let it preheat.

2. Meanwhile, take a medium bowl, place flours in it, and stir in the baking powder until mixed.

3.   Add eggs along with sour cream and oil, whisk until blended and then fold in cheese, tomato, and olives until just mixed.

4.   Take two silicone muffin cups, add the prepared batter in it evenly and then bake for 10 to 12 minutes until cooked but slightly moist in the middle.

5.   When done, let muffin cools for 5 minutes, then take them out and serve.

Nutrition: 256 Calories; 23.5 g Fats; 8.7 g Protein; 1 g Net Carb; 1.8 g Fiber;

Green Beans with Herbs

Preparation time: 5 minutes

Cooking time: 7 minutes

Servings: 2

Ingredients:

- 3 oz green beans
- 2 slices of bacon, diced
- 3 tbsp chopped parsley
- 3 tbsp chopped cilantro
- tbsp avocado oil
- Seasoning:
- ½ tsp garlic powder
- ¼ tsp salt

Directions:

1. Place green beans in a medium heatproof bowl, cover with a plastic wrap, and then microwave for 3 to 4 minutes at high heat setting until tender.

2. Meanwhile, take a medium skillet pan, place it over medium heat and when hot, add bacon and cook for 3 to 4 minutes until crisp.

3.   Season bacon with salt, sprinkle with garlic powder and cook for 30 seconds until fragrant, remove the pan from heat.

4.   When green beans have steamed, drain them well, rinse under cold water, and then transfer to a bowl.

5.   Add bacon and remaining ingredients and toss until well mixed.

6.   Serve.

Nutrition: 380 Calories; 33.7 g Fats; 15.2 g Protein; 2.4 g Net Carb; 1.4 g Fiber;

Paprika 'n Cajun Seasoned Onion Rings

Preparation Time: 15 minutes

Cooking Time: 25 minutes

Servings: 6

Ingredients:

- large white onion
- large eggs, beaten
- ½ teaspoon Cajun seasoning
- ¾ cup almond flour
- ½ teaspoon paprika
- ½ cups coconut oil for frying
- ¼ cup water
- Salt and pepper to taste

Directions:

1. Preheat a pot with oil for 8 minutes.

2. Peel the onion cut off the top and slice into circles.

3. In a mixing bowl, combine the water and the eggs.

Season with pepper and salt.

4. Soak the onion in the egg mixture.

5.   In another bowl, combine the almond flour, paprika powder, Cajun seasoning, salt, and pepper.

6.   Dredge the onion in the almond flour mixture.

7.   Place in the pot and cook in batches until golden brown, around 8 minutes per batch.

Nutrition: Calories: 262 Fat: 24.1g Carbs: 3.9g Protein: 2.8g

SOUP AND STEWS

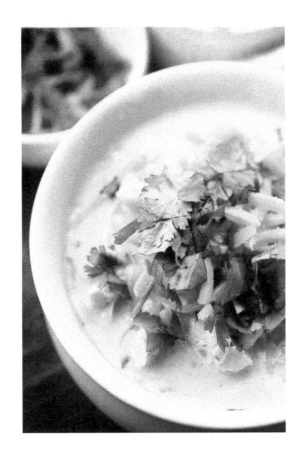

Cheesy Tomato And Basil Soup

Preparation time: 5 minutes

Cooking time: 15 minutes

Servings: 12

Ingredients:

- 2 (14 ounces / 397 g) canned whole tomatoes, diced

- tablespoon dried basil

- tablespoons coconut oil

- ounces (113 g) red onions, finely diced

- teaspoon dried oregano

- garlic cloves, minced

- 8 ounces (227 g) cream cheese, softened

- cups chicken broth

- ounces (142 g) grated Parmesan cheese, plus more for garnishing

- teaspoon salt

- ¼ teaspoon ground black pepper

- Fresh basil, chopped, for garnishing

Directions:

1.   Grease a nonstick skillet with coconut oil, and sauté the onions, basil, oregano, and garlic in the skillet for 4 minutes or until aromatic.

2.   Put in the cream cheese and fully whisk until no clump, then fold in the chicken broth, and put in the cheese, tomatoes, salt, and pepper. Stir to combine well.

3.   Cover the lid and bring them to a simmer over medium heat for 8 minutes. Transfer the soup into a blender, then blitz until thickened.

4.   Gently pour the soup into a large serving bowl and scatter with Parmesan cheese and basil as garnish.

Nutrition: calories: 146 total fat: 12g net carbs: 3g fiber: 1g protein: 6g

Chicken And Cauliflower Curry Stew

Preparation time: 15 minutes

Cooking time: 4 hours

Servings: 7

Ingredients:

o   pounds (680 g) skinless, boneless chicken thighs, cut into bite-sized pieces

•   pound (454 g) cauliflower, chopped into small pieces

•   ⅓ cup coconut oil

•   tablespoons ginger garlic paste

•   tablespoons curry powder

•   Salt and ground black pepper, to taste

•   green bell pepper, chopped

•   14 ounces (397 g) unsweetened coconut milk

•   ¼ cup fresh cilantro, chopped

Directions:

1.   Warm half of the coconut oil in a nonstick skillet over medium heat, then sauté the garlic ginger paste and curry powder for 1 minutes or until aromatic.

2.   Put in the chicken pieces, and sprinkle with salt and pepper. sauté for an additional 10 minutes or until the chicken is lightly browned. Remove from the skillet and set aside in warm.

3.   Warm another half of coconut oil in the skillet, then sauté the cauliflower and bell pepper over medium-high heat for 1 to 2 minutes.

4.   Then fold in the coconut milk and lower the heat to low. Cover with lid and stew for 45 minutes.

5.   Sprinkle with salt and pepper, then put in the sautéed chicken. Transfer the stew to a large platter and serve with cilantro on top as garnish.

Nutrition: calories: 782 total fat: 68g net carbs: 9g fiber: 5g protein: 33g

Roasted Garlic Lemon Dip

Preparation Time: 5 minutes

Cooking Time: 30 minutes

Servings: 3

Ingredients:

- 3 medium lemons

- 3 cloves garlic, peeled and smashed

- 5 tablespoons olive oil, divided

- 1/2 teaspoon kosher salt

- Pepper to taste

- Salt

- Pepper

Directions:

1.   Bring the rack in the center of the oven then heat to 400°F.

2.   Cut the lemons in half crosswise and take off the seeds. Put the lemons cut-side up in a small baking dish. Add the garlic and drizzle with 2 tablespoons of the oil.

3.   Roast until the lemons are tender and lightly browned, about 30 minutes. Take off the baking dish to a wire rack.

4.   Once the lemons are cool enough to handle, squeeze the juice into the baking dish. Discard the lemon pieces and any remaining seeds. Put the contents of the baking dish, including the garlic, into a blender or mini food processor. Put the remaining 3 tablespoons oil and salt. Process until the garlic is completely puréed, and the sauce is emulsified and slightly thickened. Serve warm or at room temperature.

Nutrition: Calories: 165 Fat: 17g Carbs: 4.8g Protein: 0.6g

DESSERT

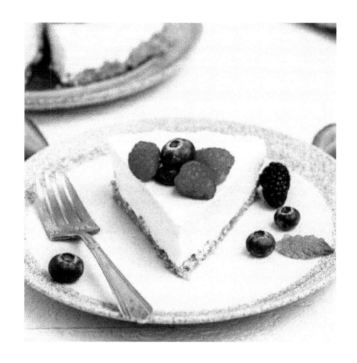

Cinnamon and Cardamom Fat Bombs

Preparation Time: 12 minutes

Cooking Time: 45 minutes

Servings: 10

Ingredients:

- Unsalted butter 3 oz.
- Unsweetened finely shredded coconut 1/2 cup
- Ground cardamom (green) 1 tsp.
- Ground cinnamon 1 tsp.
- Vanilla extract 1/2 tsp.

Directions

1. Bring butter to room temperature.

2. Carefully roast the shredded coconut over medium heat, until finely browned. It will produce a wonderful taste, but if you want to, you can skip this.

3. In a bowl, add butter, half the shredded coconut, and spices. Chill mixture for 5-10 minutes in a fridge until somewhat solid.

4.	Shape into small balls. Roll balls into remaining shredded coconut.

5.	Keep in the fridge or freezer.

Nutrition: Calories 139 Total Fat 4.6 g Total Carbs 2.5 g Sugar 6.3 g Fiber 0.6 g Protein 3.8 g

Keto Tres Leches Cake

Preparation Time: 12 minutes

Cooking Time: 65 minutes

Servings: 8

Ingredients:

- Cake

- Eggs 3

- Almond flour 31/2 oz.

- Coconut flour 1 tbsp.

- Whipping cream 2 tbsp.

- Baking powder 1 tsp.

- Tartar cream 1/2 tsp.

- Unsalted butter for greasing the baking dish

- Erythritol 31/2 oz.

- Sauce

- Whipping cream 1/2 cup

- Almond milk unsweetened 1/2 cup

- Erythritol powdered 21/2 tbsp.

- Vanilla extract 1 tbsp.

- Salt 1 pinch

- Xanthan gum 1/4 tsp.

- Cream

- Whipping cream 1/2 cup

- Cream cheese at room temperature 1 tsp.

- Powdered erythritol 2 tsp.

- To serve

- Ground cinnamon 1 tsp.

Directions:

1. Combine all ingredients in a bowl. Mix well until mixed.

2. Grease a 16 x 21 cm (6 "x 9") glass baking platter or at least 6.5 cm 2.5 " wide microwave-proof oven.

3. Place the batter into the bowl, smoothing the surface to ensure that the mixture is uniform.

4. Remove from the microwave oven. Verify if the cake in the middle is cooked. If possible, return to the microwave oven for 20 secs. Continue this phase until the cake middle is cooked at room temperature, allowing to cool it and don't remove from the microwave oven, the cake. Continue this method until the cake center is cooked.

5.   Mix the ingredients for the sauce as the cake is cooling in the oven, then mix until dissolves the erythritol. Place on aside.

6.   Assembly

7.   Using a fork to poke uniformly spaced holes over the cake top. Pour the sauce all over the cake top. Refrigerate for 2 hours at least or overnight, so that the sauce is consumed by the dish.

8.   Combine the whipped cream ingredients and with an electric mixer, beat until the mixture creates peaks (about 2 minutes). Be cautious not to beat faster than enough, or it will transform into butter.

9.   Cover with the whipped cream around the sandwich. Just before eating, sprinkle with ground cinnamon.

Nutrition: Calories 136 Total Fat 10.7 g Total Carbs 1.2 g Sugar 1.4 g Fiber 0.2 g Protein 0.9

Keto goat cheese with blackberries and roasted pistachios

Preparation Time: 12 minutes

Cooking Time: 72 minutes

Servings: 4

Ingredients:

- Goat cheese 20 oz.

- Blackberry sauce

- Fresh blackberries 9 oz.

- Erythritol 1 tbsp.

- Ground cinnamon 1 pinch

- Topping

- Pistachio nuts 1 oz.

- Salt

- Fresh rosemary

Instructions

1. To 350F preheat the oven.

2. Combine blackberries, cinnamon, and sweetener, if using. Set aside.

3.   Bake the goat cheese in the oven for about 10 to 12 minutes or until it gets some color. Remove and let sit for a few minutes.

4.   Roughly chop the pistachios and roast them in a dry frying pan. Season with salt.

5.   Top the goat cheese with blackberry, roasted pistachio, and rosemary.

Nutrition: Calories 252 Total Fat 17.3 g Total Carbs 3.2 g Sugar 0.3 g Fiber 1.4 g Protein 5.2 g

Keto Argentine Cookie and Caramel Sandwiches

Preparation Time: 12 minutes

Cooking Time: 65 minutes

Servings: 8

Ingredients:

- Butter 1 cup

- Erythritol 1/3 cup

- Vanilla extract 1 tsp.

- Salt 1 pinch

- 2 cups fine ground, blanched almond flour

- Butter or ghee 2 tbsp.

- Heavy whipping cream or coconut cream 1/3 cup

- Erythritol 1/2 cup

- Nut butter 1 tbsp.

Directions:

1.   In a large bowl, beat butter and sweetener until smooth.

2.   Add in the vanilla and salt and beat to combine.

3.   Add in the almond flour and mix until well incorporated, then use a spatula to smooth it out.

4.   Transfer the dough to a piece of parchment paper and roll it into a log.

5.   Wrap it up and let cool in the fridge to harden for one hour. In the meantime, let's prepare the caramel.

6.   In a small saucepot or skillet on medium heat, melt the butter or ghee until browned.

7.   Add in cream and sweetener and bring to a simmer.

8.   Reduce heat to medium-low and occasionally stir until the sweetener is dissolved and the liquid is thick and sticky and easily coats a spoon inserted in the mix.

9.   Remove from the heat and transfer it to a jar and let it cool at room temperature.

10.   Stir it as it cools every few minutes to make sure it does not separate.

11.   If your caramel does not thicken enough to spread on the cookies, mix in the nut butter.

12.   Preheat the oven to 325°F (160°C).

13.   Line a sheet pan with parchment paper.

14. Cut 1/4 inch thick rounds of dough and lay each slice carefully on the sheet pan, using your fingers to shape the cookie to an even round shape with smooth edges. Make 12 cookies. You need an even number for the sandwiches.

15. Leave 1-2 inches (3-5 cm) between them and bake for 15 minutes or until the edges are golden brown.

16. Remove from the oven and let them cool before transferring to a wire rack.

17. When the cookies are room temperature, turn them over.

18. Add a heaping tablespoon of caramel to every other cookie, then top the sandwich, gently pressing down until the spread reaches the edges.

Nutrition: Calories 136 Total Fat 10.7 g Total Carbs 1.2 g Sugar 1.4 g Fiber 0.2 g Protein 0.9

Cocoa Keto cookies

Preparation time: 10 minutes

Cooking time: 15 minutes

Servings 11

Ingredients:

- 1/2 Cup of Swerve confectioner

- 1/2 Cup of Unsweetened Cocoa Powder

- 4 Tablespoons of almond butter

- 2 Large Eggs

- 1 Teaspoon of vanilla extract

- 1 Cup of Almond Flour

- 1 Teaspoon of baking powder

- 1 Pinch of Pink Salt

Directions:

1.   Combine the cocoa powder with the swerve in a large mixing bowl; then add then add the melted butter to the mixture and combine all together with the help of a hand mixer.

2.   Once your ingredients are very well combined, add the eggs, the vanilla, and the baking powder and mix again.

3. Add in the almond flour and mix again; the batter should be thick.

4. Form cookies from the dough and arrange it over a baking sheet.

5. Bake your cookies for about 13 to 14 minutes at a temperature if about 350 F.

6. Serve and enjoy your cookies or store them in a clean container to serve whenever you want!

Nutrition: Calories: 16 Fat: 17.4 g Carbohydrates: 2.5g Fiber: 1gProtein: 4

Brownie cookies

Preparation time: 20 minutes

Cooking time: 10 minutes

Servings 11

Ingredients:

- 2 Tablespoons of softened almond butter

- 1 Large egg

- 1 Tablespoon of Truvia

- 1/4 Cup of Splenda

- 1/8 Teaspoon of blackstrap molasses

- 1 Tablespoon of vita fiber syrup

- 1 Teaspoon of vanilla extract

- 6 Tablespoon of sugar-free chocolate-chips

- 1 Teaspoon of almond butter

- 6 Tablespoons of almond flour

- 1 Tablespoon of cocoa powder

- 1/8 Teaspoon of baking powder

- 1/8 Teaspoon of salt

- 1/4 Teaspoon of xanthan gum

- 1/4 Cup of chopped pecans

- 1 Tablespoon of sugar-free chocolate-chips

Directions:

1.   In a medium bowl, and with a hand mixer, mix all together two tablespoons of almond butter with the egg, the sweeteners, the vita fiber and the vanilla and combine for about 2 minutes.

2.   In a separate medium bowl, microwave the chocolate chips and about 1 tablespoon of the almond butter for about 30 seconds.

3.   Beat the chocolate into the mixture of eggs and butter and mix until you get a smooth batter.

4.   Stir in the remaining almond flour, the cocoa powder, the baking powder, the salt, the xanthan gum, the chopped pecans and the chocolate chips.

5.   Place the batter in the freezer for about 7 to 8 minutes to firm up; then preheat your oven to about 350 F.

6. Spray a large baking sheet with oil and make the shape of cookies with your hands.

7. Arrange the cookies over the baking sheet and lightly flatten each of the cookies with your hand or with the back of an oiled spoon.

8. Bake your cookies for about 8 to 10min.

9. Let the cookies rest for about 10 minutes to cool.

10. Serve and enjoy your delicious cookies!

Nutrition: Calories: 61 Fat: 4 g Carbohydrates: 3g Fiber: 0.9g Protein: 1.2

Lightning Source UK Ltd.
Milton Keynes UK
UKHW020722270521
384465UK00005B/101